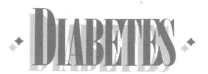

WHAT IS DIABETES?

When you have diabetes, your body can't use the food you eat in the proper way. When you eat, food is digested and much of it is changed into glucose, a sugar the body uses for fuel. The glucose is carried by the bloodstream to the individual cells of the body. The body produces a hormone called insulin that helps the glucose enter the cells. Normally, enough insulin is produced to allow the amount of glucose in the blood to be absorbed by the cells, where it is used for energy. Insulin also helps the body to store extra glucose and fat for later use.

When you have diabetes, your body does not make enough insulin or does not use it properly. Without insulin, your body cannot use the food you eat. The digested food, in the form of glucose, builds up in your blood. The cells can't get the energy they need, because insulin isn't available to move the glucose into the cells. The symptoms of diabetes are caused by high blood glucose. People with diabetes may also have high blood-fat levels (cholesterol and triglycerides). Over time, higher than normal blood-glucose and blood-fat levels may cause serious long-term complications.

There are two major types of diabetes mellitus:

- insulin-dependent (IDDM, Type I, juvenile-onset)
- non-insulin-dependent (NIDDM, Type II, adult-onset)

People with **insulin-dependent diabetes** do not make insulin. When the body has no insulin and cannot use glucose for energy, it begins to burn fat. When fat is burned for energy, acid wastes called ketones are formed. The ketones build up in the blood and cause a serious condition called ketoacidosis. People with insulin-dependent diabetes must take insulin injections to avoid this life-threatening condition.

People with **non-insulin-dependent diabetes** make some insulin, but either there is not enough insulin, or it is not working properly. People often can control this type of diabetes by limiting the amount of food they eat and by increasing their exercise. Oral hypoglycemic agents (diabetes pills) help some people to make more insulin or to use their own insulin better. Some people with non-insulin-dependent diabetes may need insulin injections to regulate their blood-glucose levels.

HOW IS DIABETES MANAGED?

The management of diabetes has three parts:

- food
- activity
- medication (if needed)

Food raises blood-glucose and blood-fat levels. Activity and medications (insulin or oral hypoglycemic agents) lower blood-glucose and blood-fat levels. A balance of these three parts leads to good management of your diabetes.

There are three nutritional goals of diabetes management:

■ **Appropriate blood-glucose and blood-fat levels.** You will learn to balance the food you eat with your activity level, and with the insulin in your body, so that your blood glucose and blood fats (cholesterol and triglycerides) stay as close to normal as possible. It is important to keep blood glucose near normal to prevent problems that can result from too high a level (ketoacidosis or diabetic coma), or if using insulin, too low a level (insulin reactions). It is important to match the amount of food you eat with the amount of insulin in your body, whether your body still produces insulin on its own or with the help of diabetes pills, or if your insulin comes from injections. This will help you to feel better—the symptoms of diabetes should disappear—but more important, it may help to reduce or prevent the complications of diabetes.

Blood-glucose monitoring can be very useful in keeping track of your diabetes, and can show you the effects of certain foods or activities on your blood-glucose levels. You can measure your own blood glucose using a finger-stick device and test strip. Your monitoring record will help you match your meal plan to other aspects of your diabetes management.

It is also important to limit the amount of fat in your diet, because high levels of blood fats are associated with heart disease. People with diabetes run a greater risk of developing heart disease than other people.

■ **Reasonable weight.** It is important to eat the right amount of calories to help you reach and stay at a reasonable body weight. The amount of calories you need depends on your size, age, and activity level. Eating the right number of calories is important for many reasons.

■ **Eating too many calories** causes weight gain, which will worsen diabetes and increase your risks for high blood pressure and heart disease. Your body makes and/or uses insulin best when you are at your desirable weight.

■ **Eating too few calories** causes a different problem. Children and teens with diabetes must eat enough calories to grow properly. Pregnant and nursing women must eat enough calories to provide for proper development of their babies.

Exercise is very important, too. It is helpful while trying to lose weight, and it is also good for your heart and blood vessels. You can increase your activity level by walking, biking, or just taking the stairs instead of an elevator. If you wish to begin an exercise training program, check with your health care team first.

■ **Good nutrition.** It is important to eat a variety of food each day. Your body works better if you eat a balanced diet that includes the right amounts of vitamins, minerals, carbohydrate, protein, and fat. Carbohydrate is the major source of energy. Protein builds muscle and tissue and provides some energy. Fat is the storage form of energy. Most foods contain a mixture of these. Carbohydrate has four calories per gram of weight, and is found in starches, bread, fruit, vegetables, and milk. Protein also has four calories per gram of weight. Protein is found in meat and milk, and small amounts of protein are found in starches, bread, and vegetables. Fat is higher in calories—nine calories per gram of weight. Fat is found in meat, dairy products, oils, and nuts. Insulin is needed to use carbohydrate, protein, and fat properly.

Here are some principles of good nutrition:

■ **Eat less fat.** The average American adult eats too much fat. Too much fat may cause heart and blood vessel disease. Eat fish, poultry, and other lean meats. Watch your portion sizes of all meat—it's easy to eat too much. Eat fewer high-fat foods such as cold cuts, bacon, nuts, gravy, salad dressing, margarine, and solid shortening. Drink skim or lowfat milk and eat less ice cream, butter, and cheese.

■ **Eat more carbohydrates (starches and breads), especially those high in fiber.** Carbohydrate foods are a good source of energy, vitamins, and minerals. Fiber in foods may help to lower blood-glucose and blood-fat levels. All people should increase the amount of carbohydrate and fiber they eat. This can be done by eating more dried beans, peas, and lentils; more whole grain breads, cereals, and crackers; and more fruit and vegetables. Foods that are high in fiber are noted in this booklet with a special symbol: .

■ **Eat less sugar.** All people, including those with diabetes, should eat less sugar. Sugar has lots of calories and no vitamins or minerals, and it causes dental cavities. Foods high in sugar include: desserts such as frosted cake and pie, sugary breakfast foods, table sugar, honey, and syrup. One 12-ounce can of regular soft drink has nine teaspoons of sugar!

■ **Use less salt.** Most of us eat too much salt. The sodium in salt can cause the body to retain water, and in some people it may raise blood pressure. High blood pressure is made worse by eating too much salt and sodium. Try to use less salt in cooking and at the table. Foods that are high in sodium, such as processed and convenience foods, are noted in this booklet with special symbols: , ★.

■ **Use alcohol in moderation.** It is best to avoid alcohol altogether. If you like to have an alcoholic drink now and then, ask your dietitian how to work it into your meal plan. If you take insulin, it is important to eat food with your drink.

How can I accomplish these goals?

A diabetes meal plan and the exchange lists will help you to meet all these goals. The first step is to talk to your dietitian, who will determine your daily nutritional needs and help you work out your own nutritional prescription. This prescription will match the calories, carbohydrate, protein, and fat you eat with your own activity level, and with the insulin in your body.

What is a diabetes meal plan?

You and your dietitian will work out a specific meal plan for you. Your meal plan is a guide which shows the number of food choices (exchanges) you can eat at each meal and snack. Your meal plan is designed so that you will eat more than half of your total daily calories as carbohydrate, and you will eat less fat and protein.

What are exchange lists?

The six exchange lists help to make your meal plan work. Foods are grouped together on a list because they are alike. Every food on a list has about the same amount of carbohydrate, protein, fat, and calories. In the amounts given, all the choices on each list are equal. Any food on a list can be exchanged or traded for any other food on the same list.

The six lists are: starch/bread, meat and substitutes, vegetables, fruit, milk, and fat.

Using the exchange lists and following your meal plan will provide you with a great variety of food choices, and will control the distribution of calories, carbohydrate, protein, and fat throughout the day, so that your food and your insulin will be balanced. This balance is what gives you good blood-glucose control.

Is the meal plan different for the different types of diabetes?

Yes, it is. The goals of treatment are somewhat different for the two types of diabetes.

Insulin-Dependent Diabetes. The most important nutrition principle for people with insulin-dependent diabetes is consistency. Meals should be eaten at about the same time each day. The amounts and types of food eaten at each meal should be about the same from day to day. This is important because the food you eat is planned to balance your insulin injections and your activity. Your meal plan and the exchange lists can help you to be consistent, so that your food and insulin work together to regulate your blood-glucose levels. If your meal plan and your insulin are out of balance, wide swings in blood glucose can occur. You may suffer from insulin reactions or from the symptoms of high blood glucose.

Non-Insulin-Dependent Diabetes. Most people with non-insulin-dependent diabetes are over-weight. Thus, the most important nutrition principle for people with this type of diabetes is weight control. You can lose weight by eating less food and increasing your exercise. It is still important to eat a balanced diet, even while losing weight. Your dietitian will help you determine the number of calories you need and set weight goals and give you tips to help you reach those goals.

Do I have to change the way I now eat?

You may have to change the way you eat. Many people ask if they can eat the same food as the rest of their family. The diabetes meal plan is not much different from the way everyone should eat. However, it is true that many people do not eat in such a healthy way. And it's very hard to change habits, especially about food. Just remember—make changes gradually, set short-term goals, and reward yourself when you are successful.

To make your meal plan work, you will need to eat what is prescribed for you. Serving sizes are very important to the success of your meal plan. If you eat too much food or too little food, your blood-glucose regulation and your weight will be affected. To help you estimate serving sizes accurately, you will need to measure or weigh your

food for the first week or so, and again periodically as time goes on to see how you're doing. Suggestions for how to measure your serving sizes are included in the "Management Tips" section of this booklet (see page 25).

It is very important to see your dietitian regularly when you are first learning how to use your meal plan and the exchange lists. Your meal plan can be adjusted if it is not working out for you. The only way to make it right is to see your dietitian and solve the problems.

Will this meal plan always be right for me?

Your meal plan may need to be changed as time goes on. Changes in lifestyle such as work, school, vacation or travel require adjustments in your meal plan. Your weight may change, your eating habits may change, your activity may change—any of these changes means you may need a new meal plan. As children grow they need more calories, and when they reach adulthood they need fewer. Check in with your dietitian regularly to review your meal plan, ask any questions you may have, and learn about new nutrition information. Regular nutrition counseling can help you make positive changes in your eating habits.

Remember, your meal plan is written just for you—it takes your likes and dislikes into consideration. It is flexible and can be adjusted for your varying needs. It is intended to help you achieve your nutrition goals. You can change your eating habits, and you'll feel better and be healthier, too. Good luck and good eating with *Exchange Lists for Meal Planning*!

EXCHANGE LISTS

The reason for dividing food into six different groups is that foods vary in their carbohydrate, protein, fat, and calorie content. Each exchange list contains foods that are alike—each choice contains about the same amount of carbohydrate, protein, fat, and calories.

The following chart shows the amount of these nutrients in one serving from each exchange list.

Exchange List	Carbohydrate (grams)	Protein (grams)	Fat (grams)	Calories
Starch/Bread	15	3	trace	80
Meat				
Lean	—	7	3	55
Medium-Fat	—	7	5	75
High-Fat	—	7	8	100
Vegetable	5	2	—	25
Fruit	15	—	—	60
Milk				
Skim	12	8	trace	90
Lowfat	12	8	5	120
Whole	12	8	8	150
Fat	—	—	5	45

As you read the exchange lists, you will notice that one choice often is a larger amount of food than another choice from the same list. Because foods are so different, each food is measured or weighed so the amount of carbohydrate, protein, fat, and calories is the same in each choice.

You will notice symbols on some foods in the exchange groups. Foods that are high in fiber (3 grams or more per exchange) have a green 🌾 symbol. High-fiber foods are good for you. It is important to eat more of these foods.

Foods that are high in sodium (400 milligrams or more of sodium per exchange) have a red 🥫 symbol; foods that have 400 mg or more of sodium if two or more exchanges are eaten have a blue ★ symbol. It's a good idea to limit your intake of high-salt foods, especially if you have high blood pressure.

If you have a favorite food that is not included in any of these groups, ask your dietitian about it. That food can probably be worked into your meal plan, at least now and then.

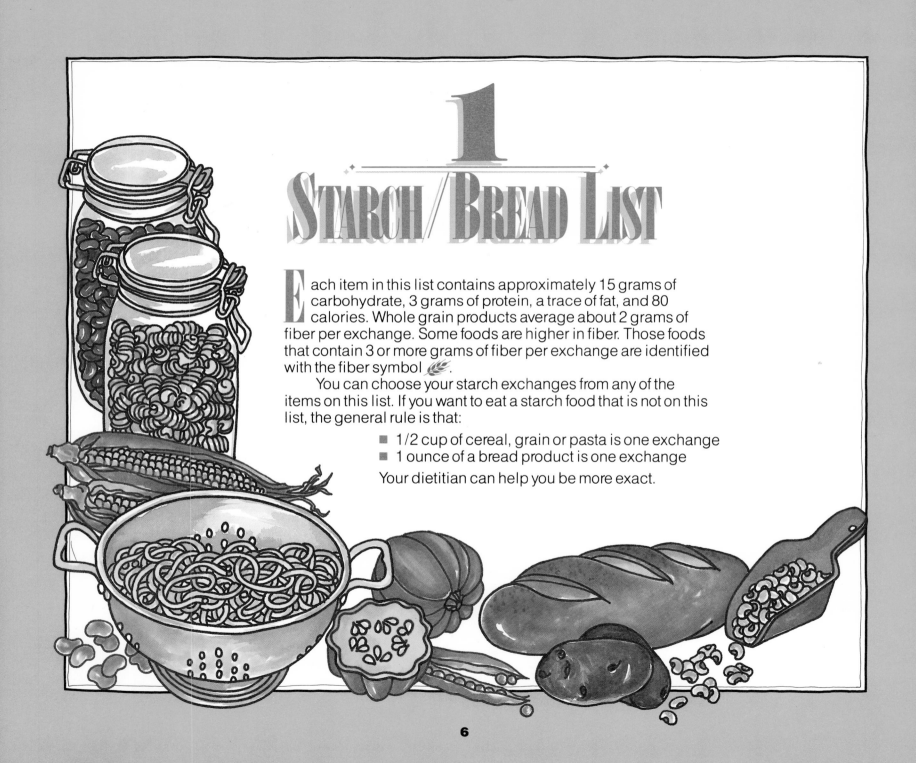

1
STARCH/BREAD LIST

E ach item in this list contains approximately 15 grams of carbohydrate, 3 grams of protein, a trace of fat, and 80 calories. Whole grain products average about 2 grams of fiber per exchange. Some foods are higher in fiber. Those foods that contain 3 or more grams of fiber per exchange are identified with the fiber symbol 🌾.

You can choose your starch exchanges from any of the items on this list. If you want to eat a starch food that is not on this list, the general rule is that:

- 1/2 cup of cereal, grain or pasta is one exchange
- 1 ounce of a bread product is one exchange

Your dietitian can help you be more exact.

CEREALS/GRAINS/PASTA

🌾 Bran cereals, concentrated (such as Bran Buds®, All Bran®)	1/3 cup
🌾 Bran cereals, flaked	1/2 cup
Bulgur (cooked)	1/2 cup
Cooked cereals	1/2 cup
Cornmeal (dry)	2 1/2 Tbsp.
Grape-Nuts®	3 Tbsp.
Grits (cooked)	1/2 cup
Other ready-to-eat unsweetened cereals	3/4 cup
Pasta (cooked)	1/2 cup
Puffed cereal	1 1/2 cup
Rice, white or brown (cooked)	1/3 cup
Shredded wheat	1/2 cup
🌾 Wheat germ	3 Tbsp.

DRIED BEANS/PEAS/LENTILS

🌾 Beans and peas (cooked) (such as kidney, white, split, blackeye)	1/3 cup
🌾 Lentils (cooked)	1/3 cup
🌾 Baked beans	1/4 cup

STARCHY VEGETABLES

🌾 Corn	1/2 cup
🌾 Corn on cob, 6 in. long	1
🌾 Lima beans	1/2 cup
🌾 Peas, green (canned or frozen)	1/2 cup
🌾 Plantain	1/2 cup
Potato, baked	1 small (3 oz.)
Potato, mashed	1/2 cup
🌾 Squash, winter (acorn, butternut)	1 cup
Yam, sweet potato, plain	1/3 cup

BREAD

Bagel	1/2 (1 oz.)
Bread sticks, crisp, 4 in. long × 1/2 in.	2 (2/3 oz.)
Croutons, lowfat	1 cup
English muffin	1/2
Frankfurter or hamburger bun	1/2 (1 oz.)
Pita, 6 in. across	1/2
Plain roll, small	1 (1 oz.)
Raisin, unfrosted	1 slice (1 oz.)
Rye, pumpernickel	1 slice (1 oz.)
Tortilla, 6 in. across	1
White (including French, Italian)	1 slice (1 oz.)
Whole wheat	1 slice (1 oz.)

🌾 *3 grams or more of fiber per exchange*

CRACKERS/SNACKS

Animal crackers	8
Graham crackers, 2 1/2 in. square	3
Matzoh	3/4 oz.
Melba toast	5 slices
Oyster crackers	24
Popcorn (popped, no fat added)	3 cups
Pretzels	3/4 oz.
🌾 Rye crisp, 2 in. × 3 1/2 in.	4
Saltine-type crackers	6
🌾 Whole-wheat crackers, no fat added (crisp breads, such as Finn®, Kavli®, Wasa®)	2-4 slices (3/4 oz.)

Taco shell, 6 in. across	2
Waffle, 4 1/2 in. square	1
🌾 Whole-wheat crackers, fat added (such as Triscuit®)	4-6 (1 oz.)

STARCH FOODS PREPARED WITH FAT

(Count as 1 starch/bread exchange, plus 1 fat exchange.)

Biscuit, 2 1/2 in. across	1
Chow mein noodles	1/2 cup
Corn bread, 2 in. cube	1 (2 oz.)
Cracker, round butter type	6
French fried potatoes, 2 in. to 3 1/2 in. long	10 (1 1/2 oz.)
Muffin, plain, small	1
Pancake, 4 in. across	2
Stuffing, bread (prepared)	1/4 cup

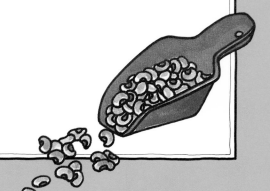

2
MEAT LIST

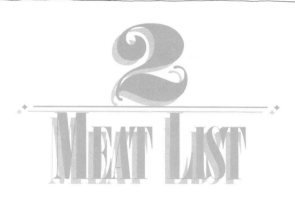

Each serving of meat and substitutes on this list contains about 7 grams of protein. The amount of fat and number of calories varies, depending on what kind of meat or substitute you choose. The list is divided into three parts based on the amount of fat and calories: lean meat, medium-fat meat, and high-fat meat. One ounce (one meat exchange) of each of these includes:

	Carbohydrate (grams)	Protein (grams)	Fat (grams)	Calories
Lean	0	7	3	55
Medium-Fat	0	7	5	75
High-Fat	0	7	8	100

You are encouraged to use more lean and medium-fat meat, poultry, and fish in your meal plan. This will help decrease your fat intake, which may help decrease your risk for heart disease. The items from the high-fat group are high in saturated fat, cholesterol, and calories. You should limit your choices from the high-fat group to three (3) times per week. Meat and substitutes do not contribute any fiber to your meal plan.

Meats and meat substitutes that have 400 milligrams or more of sodium per exchange are indicated with this symbol.

★ *Meats and meat substitutes that have 400 mg or more of sodium if two or more exchanges are eaten are indicated with this symbol.*

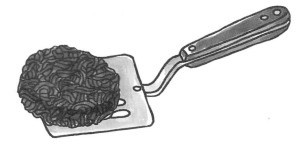

TIPS

1. Bake, roast, broil, grill, or boil these foods rather than frying them with added fat.

2. Use a nonstick pan spray or a nonstick pan to brown or fry these foods.

3. Trim off visible fat before and after cooking.

4. Do not add flour, bread crumbs, coating mixes, or fat to these foods when preparing them.

5. Weigh meat after removing bones and fat, and after cooking. Three ounces of cooked meat is about equal to 4 ounces of raw meat. Some examples of meat portions are:

2 ounces meat (2 meat exchanges) =
1 small chicken leg or thigh
1/2 cup cottage cheese or tuna

3 ounces meat (3 meat exchanges) =
1 medium pork chop
1 small hamburger
1/2 of a whole chicken breast
1 unbreaded fish fillet
cooked meat, about the size of a deck of cards

6. Restaurants usually serve prime cuts of meat, which are high in fat and calories.

LEAN MEAT AND SUBSTITUTES
(One exchange is equal to any one of the following items.)

Beef: USDA Select or Choice grades of lean beef, such as round, sirloin, and flank steak; tenderloin; and chipped beef 🥫   1 oz.

Pork: Lean pork, such as fresh ham; canned, cured or boiled ham 🥫 ; Canadian bacon 🥫 , tenderloin.   1 oz.

Veal: All cuts are lean except for veal cutlets (ground or cubed). Examples of lean veal are chops and roasts.   1 oz.

Poultry: Chicken, turkey, Cornish hen (without skin)   1 oz.

Fish:
All fresh and frozen fish   1 oz.
Crab, lobster, scallops, shrimp, clams (fresh or canned in water)   2 oz.
Oysters   6 medium
Tuna ★ (canned in water)   1/4 cup
Herring ★ (uncreamed or smoked)   1 oz.
Sardines (canned)   2 medium

Wild Game:
Venison, rabbit, squirrel   1 oz.
Pheasant, duck, goose (without skin)   1 oz.

Cheese:
Any cottage cheese ★   1/4 cup
Grated parmesan   2 Tbsp.
Diet cheeses 🥫 (with less than 55 calories per ounce)   1 oz.

Other:
95% fat-free luncheon meat 🥫   1 1/2 oz.
Egg whites   3 whites
Egg substitutes with less than 55 calories per 1/2 cup   1/2 cup

---

🥫 *400 mg or more of sodium per exchange*

★ *400 mg or more of sodium if two or more exchanges are eaten*

MEDIUM-FAT MEAT AND SUBSTITUTES
(One exchange is equal to any one of the following items.)

Beef: Most beef products fall into this category. Examples are: all ground beef, roast (rib, chuck, rump), steak (cubed, Porterhouse, T-bone), and meatloaf.   1 oz.

Pork: Most pork products fall into this category. Examples are: chops, loin roast, Boston butt, cutlets.   1 oz.

Lamb: Most lamb products fall into this category. Examples are: chops, leg, and roast.   1 oz.

Veal: Cutlet (ground or cubed, unbreaded)   1 oz.

Poultry: Chicken (with skin), domestic duck or goose (well drained of fat), ground turkey   1 oz.

Fish:
Tuna ★ (canned in oil and drained)   1/4 cup
Salmon ★ (canned)   1/4 cup

Cheese:
Skim or part-skim milk cheeses, such as:
Ricotta   1/4 cup
Mozzarella   1 oz.
Diet cheeses 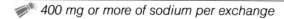 (with 56-80 calories per ounce)   1 oz.

Other:
86% fat-free luncheon meat ★   1 oz.
Egg (high in cholesterol, limit to 3 per week)   1
Egg substitutes with 56-80 calories per 1/4 cup   1/4 cup
Tofu (2 1/2 in. × 2 3/4 in. × 1 in.)   4 oz.
Liver, heart, kidney, sweetbreads   1 oz.
   (high in cholesterol)

---

 400 mg or more of sodium per exchange

★   *400 mg or more of sodium if two or more exchanges are eaten*

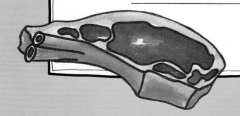

HIGH-FAT MEAT AND SUBSTITUTES

Remember, these items are high in saturated fat, cholesterol, and calories, and should be used only three (3) times per week.

(One exchange is equal to any one of the following items.)

Beef:	Most USDA Prime cuts of beef, such as ribs, corned beef ★	1 oz.
Pork:	Spareribs, ground pork, pork sausage (patty or link)	1 oz.
Lamb:	Patties (ground lamb)	1 oz.
Fish:	Any fried fish product	1 oz.
Cheese:	All regular cheeses, such as American, Blue, Cheddar ★, Monterey Jack ★, Swiss	1 oz.
Other:	Luncheon meat, such as bologna, salami, pimento loaf	1 oz.
	Sausage, such as Polish, Italian smoked	1 oz.
	Knockwurst	1 oz.
	Bratwurst ★	1 oz.
	Frankfurter (turkey or chicken)	1 frank (10/lb.)
	Peanut butter (contains unsaturated fat)	1 Tbsp.

Count as one high-fat meat plus one fat exchange:

Frankfurter (beef, pork, or combination)	1 frank (10/lb.)

---

400 mg or more of sodium per exchange

★ *400 mg or more of sodium if two or more exchanges are eaten*

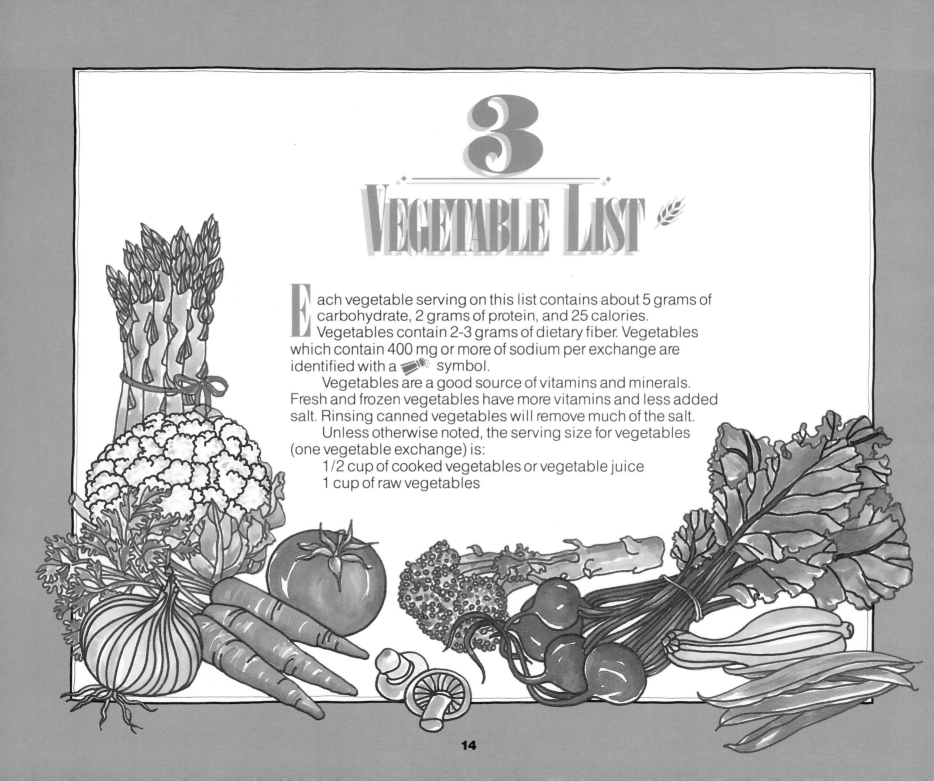

3
VEGETABLE LIST

Each vegetable serving on this list contains about 5 grams of carbohydrate, 2 grams of protein, and 25 calories.
Vegetables contain 2-3 grams of dietary fiber. Vegetables which contain 400 mg or more of sodium per exchange are identified with a 🧂 symbol.

Vegetables are a good source of vitamins and minerals. Fresh and frozen vegetables have more vitamins and less added salt. Rinsing canned vegetables will remove much of the salt.

Unless otherwise noted, the serving size for vegetables (one vegetable exchange) is:

    1/2 cup of cooked vegetables or vegetable juice
    1 cup of raw vegetables

Artichoke (1/2 medium)
Asparagus
Beans (green, wax, Italian)
Bean sprouts
Beets
Broccoli
Brussels sprouts
Cabbage, cooked
Carrots
Cauliflower
Eggplant
Greens (collard, mustard, turnip)
Kohlrabi
Leeks

Mushrooms, cooked
Okra
Onions
Pea pods
Peppers (green)
Rutabaga
Sauerkraut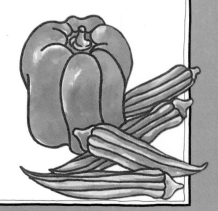
Spinach, cooked
Summer squash (crookneck)
Tomato (one large)
Tomato/vegetable juice
Turnips
Water chestnuts
Zucchini, cooked

Starchy vegetables such as corn, peas, and potatoes are found on the Starch/Bread List.

For free vegetables, see Free Food List on page 22.

---

 400 mg or more of sodium per exchange

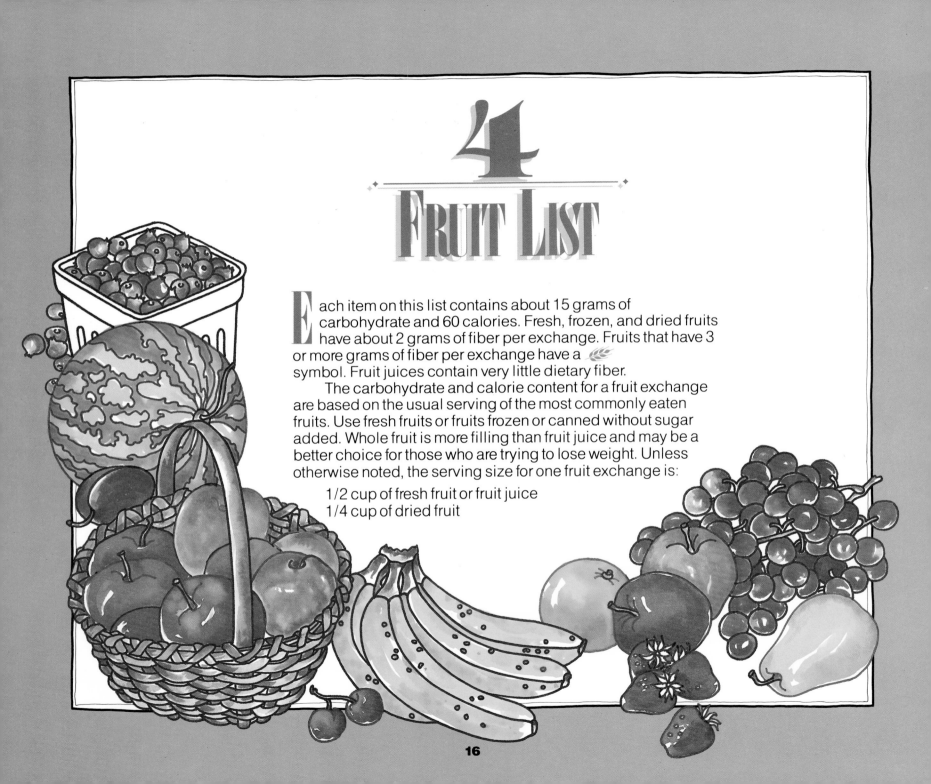

4

Fruit List

Each item on this list contains about 15 grams of carbohydrate and 60 calories. Fresh, frozen, and dried fruits have about 2 grams of fiber per exchange. Fruits that have 3 or more grams of fiber per exchange have a 🌾 symbol. Fruit juices contain very little dietary fiber.

The carbohydrate and calorie content for a fruit exchange are based on the usual serving of the most commonly eaten fruits. Use fresh fruits or fruits frozen or canned without sugar added. Whole fruit is more filling than fruit juice and may be a better choice for those who are trying to lose weight. Unless otherwise noted, the serving size for one fruit exchange is:

1/2 cup of fresh fruit or fruit juice
1/4 cup of dried fruit

FRESH, FROZEN, AND UNSWEETENED CANNED FRUIT

Apple (raw, 2 in. across)	1 apple
Applesauce (unsweetened)	1/2 cup
Apricots (medium, raw)	4 apricots
Apricots (canned)	1/2 cup, or 4 halves
Banana (9 in. long)	1/2 banana
🌾 Blackberries (raw)	3/4 cup
🌾 Blueberries (raw)	3/4 cup
Cantaloupe (5 in. across) (cubes)	1/3 melon 1 cup
Cherries (large, raw)	12 cherries
Cherries (canned)	1/2 cup
Figs (raw, 2 in. across)	2 figs
Fruit cocktail (canned)	1/2 cup
Grapefruit (medium)	1/2 grapefruit
Grapefruit (segments)	3/4 cup
Grapes (small)	15 grapes
Honeydew melon (medium) (cubes)	1/8 melon 1 cup
Kiwi (large)	1 kiwi
Mandarin oranges	3/4 cup
Mango (small)	1/2 mango
🌾 Nectarine (2 1/2 in. across)	1 nectarine
Orange (2 1/2 in. across)	1 orange
Papaya	1 cup
Peach (2 3/4 in. across)	1 peach, or 3/4 cup
Peaches (canned)	1/2 cup or 2 halves
Pear	1/2 large, or 1 small
Pears (canned)	1/2 cup, or 2 halves
Persimmon (medium, native)	2 persimmons
Pineapple (raw)	3/4 cup
Pineapple (canned)	1/3 cup
Plum (raw, 2 in. across)	2 plums
🌾 Pomegranate	1/2 pomegranate
🌾 Raspberries (raw)	1 cup
🌾 Strawberries (raw, whole)	1 1/4 cup
🌾 Tangerine (2 1/2 in. across)	2 tangerines
Watermelon (cubes)	1 1/4 cup

DRIED FRUIT

🌾 Apples	4 rings
🌾 Apricots	7 halves
Dates	2 1/2 medium
🌾 Figs	1 1/2
🌾 Prunes	3 medium
Raisins	2 Tbsp.

FRUIT JUICE

Apple juice/cider	1/2 cup
Cranberry juice cocktail	1/3 cup
Grapefruit juice	1/2 cup
Grape juice	1/3 cup
Orange juice	1/2 cup
Pineapple juice	1/2 cup
Prune juice	1/3 cup

🌾 *3 or more grams of fiber per exchange*

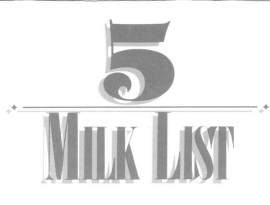

5
MILK LIST

Each serving of milk or milk products on this list contains about 12 grams of carbohydrate and 8 grams of protein. The amount of fat in milk is measured in percent (%) of butterfat. The calories vary, depending on what kind of milk you choose. The list is divided into three parts based on the amount of fat and calories: skim/very lowfat milk, lowfat milk, and whole milk. One serving (one milk exchange) of each of these includes:

	Carbohydrate (grams)	Protein (grams)	Fat (grams)	Calories
Skim/Very Lowfat	12	8	trace	90
Lowfat	12	8	5	120
Whole	12	8	8	150

Milk is the body's main source of calcium, the mineral needed for growth and repair of bones. Yogurt is also a good source of calcium. Yogurt and many dry or powdered milk products have different amounts of fat. If you have questions about a particular item, read the label to find out the fat and calorie content.

Milk is good to drink, but it can also be added to cereal, and to other foods. Many tasty dishes such as sugar-free pudding are made with milk (see the Combination Foods list). Add life to plain yogurt by adding one of your fruit exchanges to it.

SKIM AND VERY LOWFAT MILK

skim milk	1 cup
1/2% milk	1 cup
1% milk	1 cup
lowfat buttermilk	1 cup
evaporated skim milk	1/2 cup
dry nonfat milk	1/3 cup
plain nonfat yogurt	8 oz.

LOWFAT MILK

2% milk	1 cup fluid
plain lowfat yogurt (with added nonfat milk solids)	8 oz.

WHOLE MILK

The whole milk group has much more fat per serving than the skim and lowfat groups. Whole milk has more than 3 1/4% butterfat. Try to limit your choices from the whole milk group as much as possible.

whole milk	1 cup
evaporated whole milk	1/2 cup
whole plain yogurt	8 oz.

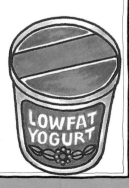

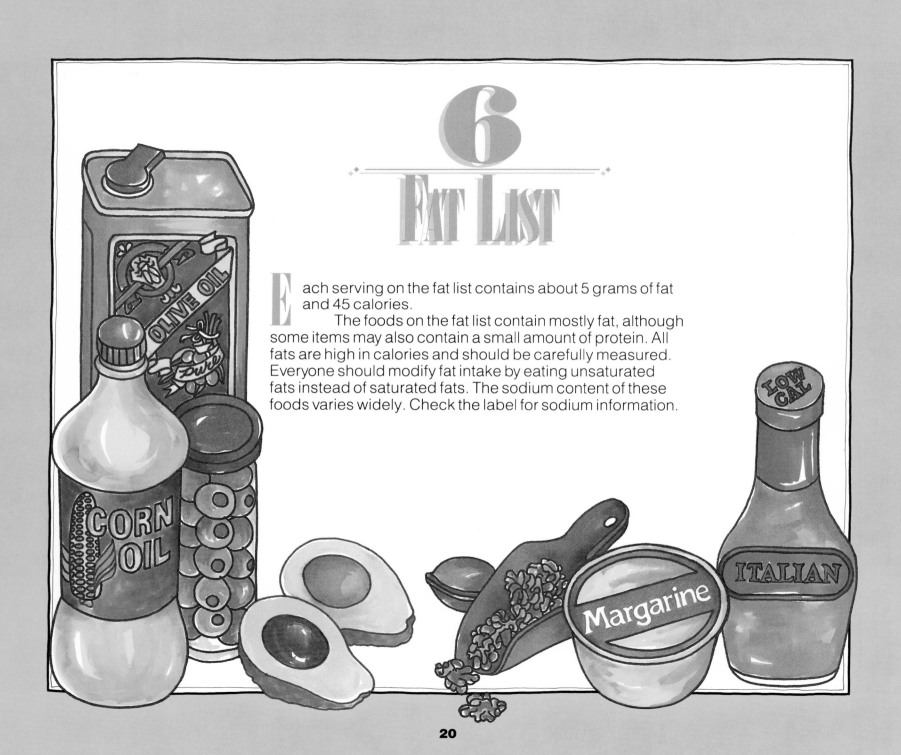

6
FAT LIST

E ach serving on the fat list contains about 5 grams of fat and 45 calories.

The foods on the fat list contain mostly fat, although some items may also contain a small amount of protein. All fats are high in calories and should be carefully measured. Everyone should modify fat intake by eating unsaturated fats instead of saturated fats. The sodium content of these foods varies widely. Check the label for sodium information.

UNSATURATED FATS

Avocado	1/8 medium
Margarine	1 tsp.
★ Margarine, diet	1 Tbsp.
Mayonnaise	1 tsp.
★ Mayonnaise, reduced-calorie	1 Tbsp.

Nuts and Seeds:

Almonds, dry roasted	6 whole
Cashews, dry roasted	1 Tbsp.
Pecans	2 whole
Peanuts	20 small or 10 large
Walnuts	2 whole
Other nuts	1 Tbsp.
Seeds, pine nuts, sun-flower (without shells)	1 Tbsp.
Pumpkin seeds	2 tsp.

Oil (corn, cottonseed, safflower, soybean, sunflower, olive, peanut)	1 tsp.
★ Olives	10 small or 5 large
Salad dressing, mayonnaise-type	2 tsp.
Salad dressing, mayonnaise-type, reduced-calorie	1 Tbsp.
★ Salad dressing (oil varieties)	1 Tbsp.

 Salad dressing, reduced-calorie — 2 Tbsp.

(Two tablespoons of low-calorie salad dressing is a free food.)

SATURATED FATS

Butter	1 tsp.
★ Bacon	1 slice
Chitterlings	1/2 ounce
Coconut, shredded	2 Tbsp.
Coffee whitener, liquid	2 Tbsp.
Coffee whitener, powder	4 tsp.
Cream (light, coffee, table)	2 Tbsp.
Cream, sour	2 Tbsp.
Cream (heavy, whipping)	1 Tbsp.
Cream cheese	1 Tbsp.
★ Salt pork	1/4 ounce

---

400 mg or more of sodium per exchange

★ *400 mg or more of sodium if two or more exchanges are eaten*

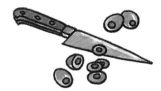

FREE FOODS

A **free food** is any food or drink that contains less than 20 calories per serving. You can eat as much as you want of those items that have no serving size specified. You may eat two or three servings per day of those items that have a specific serving size. Be sure to spread them out through the day.

Drinks:
Bouillon 🥫 or broth without fat
Bouillon, low-sodium
Carbonated drinks, sugar-free
Carbonated water
Club soda
Cocoa powder, unsweetened (1 Tbsp.)
Coffee / Tea
Drink mixes, sugar-free
Tonic water, sugar-free

Nonstick pan spray

Fruit:
Cranberries, unsweetened (1/2 cup)
Rhubarb, unsweetened (1/2 cup)

Vegetables:
(raw, 1 cup)
Cabbage
Celery
Chinese cabbage 🌾
Cucumber
Green onion
Hot peppers
Mushrooms
Radishes
Zucchini 🌾

Salad greens:
Endive
Escarole
Lettuce
Romaine
Spinach

Sweet Substitutes:
Candy, hard, sugar-free
Gelatin, sugar-free
Gum, sugar-free
Jam / Jelly, sugar-free (less than 20 cal./2 tsp.)
Pancake syrup, sugar-free (1-2 Tbsp.)

Sugar substitutes (saccharin, aspartame)
Whipped topping (2 Tbsp.)

Condiments:
Catsup (1 Tbsp.)
Horseradish
Mustard
Pickles 🥫 , dill, unsweetened
Salad dressing, low-calorie (2 Tbsp.)
Taco sauce (3 Tbsp.)
Vinegar

Seasonings can be very helpful in making food taste better. Be careful of how much sodium you use. Read the label, and choose those seasonings that do not contain sodium or salt.

Basil (fresh)
Celery seeds
Chili powder
Chives
Cinnamon
Curry
Dill

Flavoring extracts (vanilla, almond, walnut, peppermint, butter, lemon, etc.)
Garlic
Garlic powder
Herbs
Hot pepper sauce
Lemon

Lemon juice
Lemon pepper
Lime
Lime juice
Mint
Onion powder
Oregano
Paprika
Pepper

Pimento
Spices
Soy sauce 🥫
Soy sauce 🥫 , low-sodium ("lite")
Wine, used in cooking (1/4 cup)
Worcestershire sauce

🌾 *3 grams or more of fiber per exchange*   *400 mg or more of sodium per exchange*

COMBINATION FOODS

Much of the food we eat is mixed together in various combinations. These combination foods do not fit into only one exchange list. It can be quite hard to tell what is in a certain casserole dish or baked food item. This is a list of average values for some typical combination foods. This list will help you fit these foods into your meal plan. Ask your dietitian for information about any other foods you'd like to eat. The *American Diabetes Association/American Dietetic Association Family Cookbooks* and the *American Diabetes Association Holiday Cookbook* have many recipes and further information about many foods, including combination foods. Check your library or local bookstore.

Food	Amount	Exchanges
Casseroles, homemade	1 cup (8 oz.)	2 starch, 2 medium-fat meat, 1 fat
Cheese pizza 🥫, thin crust	1/4 of 15 oz. or 1/4 of 10"	2 starch, 1 medium-fat meat, 1 fat
Chili with beans 🌾, 🥫 (commercial)	1 cup (8 oz.)	2 starch, 2 medium-fat meat, 2 fat
Chow mein 🥫 (without noodles or rice)	2 cups (16 oz.)	1 starch, 2 vegetable, 2 lean meat
Macaroni and cheese 🥫	1 cup (8 oz.)	2 starch, 1 medium-fat meat, 2 fat
Soup:		
Bean 🌾, 🥫	1 cup (8 oz.)	1 starch, 1 vegetable, 1 lean meat
Chunky, all varieties 🥫	10-3/4 oz. can	1 starch, 1 vegetable, 1 medium-fat meat
Cream 🥫 (made with water)	1 cup (8 oz.)	1 starch, 1 fat
Vegetable 🥫 or broth-type 🥫	1 cup (8 oz.)	1 starch
Spaghetti and meatballs 🥫 (canned)	1 cup (8 oz.)	2 starch, 1 medium-fat meat, 1 fat
Sugar-free pudding (made with skim milk)	1/2 cup	1 starch
If beans are used as a meat substitute:		
Dried beans 🌾, peas 🌾, lentils 🌾	1 cup (cooked)	2 starch, 1 lean meat

🌾 *3 grams or more of fiber per exchange*   🥫 *400 mg or more of sodium per exchange*

FOODS FOR OCCASIONAL USE

Moderate amounts of some foods can be used in your meal plan, in spite of their sugar or fat content, as long as you can maintain blood-glucose control. The following list includes average exchange values for some of these foods. Because they are concentrated sources of carbohydrate, you will notice that the portion sizes are very small. Check with your dietitian for advice on how often and when you can eat them.

Food	Amount	Exchanges
Angel food cake	1/12 cake	2 starch
Cake, no icing	1/12 cake, or a 3" square	2 starch, 2 fat
Cookies	2 small (1 3/4" across)	1 starch, 1 fat
Frozen fruit yogurt	1/3 cup	1 starch
Gingersnaps	3	1 starch
Granola	1/4 cup	1 starch, 1 fat
Granola bars	1 small	1 starch, 1 fat
Ice cream, any flavor	1/2 cup	1 starch, 2 fat
Ice milk, any flavor	1/2 cup	1 starch, 1 fat
Sherbet, any flavor	1/4 cup	1 starch
Snack chips ★, all varieties	1 oz.	1 starch, 2 fat
Vanilla wafers	6 small	1 starch

★   *400 mg or more of sodium if two or more exchanges are eaten*

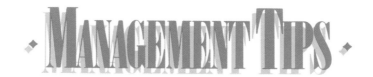
Here are some tips that can help you to change the way you eat.

■ **Make changes gradually.** Don't try to do everything all at once. It may take longer to accomplish your goals, but the changes you make will be permanent!

■ **Set short-term, realistic goals.** If weight loss is your goal, try to lose two pounds in two weeks, not 20 pounds in one week. Walk two blocks at first, not two miles. Success will come more easily, and you'll feel good about yourself!

■ **Reward yourself.** When you make your short-term goal, do something special for yourself. Go to a movie, buy a new shirt, read a book, visit a friend.

■ **Measure foods.** It is important to eat the right serving sizes of food. You will need to learn how to estimate the amount of food you are served. You can do this by measuring all the food you eat for a week or so. Measure liquids with a measuring cup. Some solid foods (tuna, cottage cheese, canned fruits) can be measured with a measuring cup, too. Measuring spoons (teaspoon, tablespoon) are used for measuring smaller amounts such as oil, salad dressing or peanut butter. A scale can be very useful to measure almost anything, especially meat, poultry and fish. All food should be measured or weighed after cooking.

Some food you buy uncooked will weigh less after you cook it. This is true of most meats. Starches often swell in cooking, so a small amount of uncooked starch will become a much larger amount of cooked food. The following table shows some of the changes:

Food (Starch Group)	Uncooked	Cooked
Oatmeal	3 level Tbsp.	1/2 cup
Cream of Wheat	2 level Tbsp.	1/2 cup
Grits	3 level Tbsp.	1/2 cup
Rice	2 level Tbsp.	1/3 cup
Spaghetti	1/4 cup	1/2 cup
Noodles	1/3 cup	1/2 cup
Macaroni	1/4 cup	1/2 cup
Dried Beans	3 Tbsp.	1/3 cup
Dried Peas	3 Tbsp.	1/3 cup
Lentils	2 Tbsp.	1/3 cup

Food (Meat Group)	Uncooked	Cooked
Hamburger	4 ounces	3 ounces
Chicken	1 small drumstick	1 ounce
	1/2 of a whole chicken breast	2 ounces

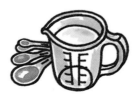

25

Read food labels. Remember dietetic does not mean diabetic! When you see the word "dietetic" on a food label, it means that something has been changed or replaced. It may have less salt, less fat, or less sugar. It does not mean that the food is sugar-free or calorie-free. Some dietetic foods may be useful. Those that contain 20 calories or less per serving may be eaten up to three times a day as free foods.

Know your sweeteners. Two types of sweeteners are on the market: those with calories and those without calories. Sweeteners with calories, such as fructose, sorbitol and mannitol, when used in large amounts may cause cramping and diarrhea. Remember, these sweeteners do have calories which add up. Sweeteners without calories include saccharin and aspartame (Equal®, NutraSweet®) and may be used in moderation.

If You Have Insulin-Dependent Diabetes:

Plan for sick days. Before you become ill with the flu or a cold, ask your doctor, dietitian, and nurse for a special sick day plan. It is important to:

- take your usual insulin dose.
- test your blood glucose regularly and check your urine for ketones.
- if you can't keep regular food down, try drinking small sips of regular soft drinks, sweetened tea, sweetened gelatin, popsicles, fruit juice, or sherbet.
- drink lots of liquids.
- call your doctor immediately if you can't keep any food down.

Prepare for insulin reactions. If you have symptoms of low blood glucose, test your blood to find out your blood-glucose level. Be sure to carry something with you at all times to treat low blood glucose. You could carry glucose tablets or hard candy.

Plan for exercise. You may need to make some changes in your meal plan or insulin dose when you begin an exercise program. Check with your dietitian or doctor about this. Be sure to carry with you some form of carbohydrate (such as dried fruit or glucose tablets) to treat low blood glucose.

Additional information on these topics is available from your dietitian or doctor.

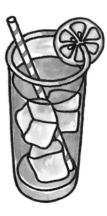

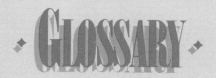

Alcohol—An ingredient in a variety of beverages, including beer, wine, liqueurs, cordials, and mixed or straight drinks. Pure alcohol itself yields about 7 calories per gram, of which more than 75% is available to the body.

Calorie—A unit used to express heat or energy value of food. Calories come from carbohydrate, protein, fat, and alcohol.

Carbohydrate—One of the three major energy sources in foods. The most common carbohydrates are sugar and starches. Carbohydrates yield about 4 calories per gram. Carbohydrates are found in foods from the milk, vegetable, fruit, and starch/bread exchange lists.

Cholesterol—A fat-like substance normally found in blood. A high level of cholesterol in the blood has been shown to be a major risk factor for developing heart disease. Dietary cholesterol is found in all animal products, but is especially high in egg yolks and organ meats. Eating foods high in dietary cholesterol and saturated fat tends to raise the level of blood cholesterol. Foods of plant origin such as fruits, vegetables, grains, and legumes contain no cholesterol. Cholesterol is found in foods from the milk, meat, and fat exchange lists.

Dietitian—a registered dietitian (R.D.) is recognized by the medical profession as the primary provider of nutritional care, education, and counseling. The initials R.D. after a dietitian's name ensure that he or she has met the standards of the American Dietetic Association. Look for this credential when you seek advice on nutrition.

Exchange—Foods grouped together on a list according to similarities in food values. Measured amount of foods within the group may be used as "trade-offs" in planning meals. A single exchange contains approximately equal amounts of carbohydrate, protein, fat, and calories.

Fat—One of the three major energy sources in food. A concentrated source of calories--about 9 calories per gram. Fat is found in foods from the fat and meat exchange lists. Some kinds of milk also have fat; some foods from the starch/bread list also contain fat.

- **Saturated fat** tends to raise blood-cholesterol levels. It comes primarily from animals and is often hard at room temperature. Examples of saturated fats are butter, lard, meat fat, solid shortening, palm oil, and coconut oil.

- **Unsaturated fat** tends to lower blood-cholesterol levels. It comes from plants and is usually liquid at room temperature. Examples of unsaturated fats are vegetable oils such as corn, cottonseed, sunflower, safflower, soybean, olive, and peanut oil.

Fiber—An indigestible part of certain foods. Fiber is important in the diet as roughage, or bulk. Fiber is found in foods from the starch/bread, vegetable, and fruit exchange lists.

- **Soluble fiber** has high water-holding capability and turns to gel during digestion. This slows digestion and the rate of nutrient absorption from the stomach and intestine. This type of fiber is found in oat bran, pectins (from fruits and vegetables) and various "gums" which are found in nuts, seeds, and legumes such as beans, lentils, and peas. This type of fiber may play a role in smoothing out the glycemic response of foods, and in reducing the likelihood of atherosclerosis.

- **Insoluble fiber** is found in foods such as wheat bran and other whole grains, and has poor water-holding capability. It appears to speed the passage of foods through the stomach and intestines, and increases fecal bulk. This type of fiber probably does not affect glycemic response or atherosclerosis.

Glycosylated Hemoglobin—A test that gives information about blood-glucose levels during the preceding 1-2 months. When blood glucose is above normal, the glucose changes the hemoglobin in red blood cells. These cells last for about 100 days, and they can be measured.

Gram—A unit of mass and weight in the metric system. An ounce is about 30 grams.

IDDM—Insulin-dependent diabetes mellitus. Individuals with IDDM are ketosis-prone, and will develop ketoacidosis if they do not take insulin regularly.

Insulin—A hormone made by the body that helps the body use food. Also, a commercially prepared injectable substance used by people who do not make enough of their own insulin.

Ketoacidosis—An increase in ketones in the blood causing the body's acid balance to tip. An emergency situation that may result in coma and death if untreated.

Ketone—An acid formed in the body when fats are burned for energy.

Meal Plan—A guide showing the number of food exchanges to use in each meal and snack to control distribution of carbohydrates, proteins, fats, and calories throughout the day.

Mineral—Substance essential in small amounts to build and repair body tissue and/or control functions of the body. Calcium, iron, magnesium, phosphorus, potassium, sodium, and zinc are minerals.

NIDDM—Non-insulin-dependent diabetes mellitus. Individuals with NIDDM may or may not take insulin for better control of their blood-glucose levels; however, they are not ketosis-prone.

Nutrient—Substance in food necessary for life. Carbohydrates, proteins, fats, minerals, vitamins, and water are nutrients.

Nutrition—Combination of processes by which the body receives and uses the materials necessary for maintenance of functions, for energy, and for growth and renewal of its parts.

Protein—One of the three major nutrients in food. Protein provides about 4 calories per gram. Protein is found in foods from the milk and meat exchange lists. Smaller amounts of protein are found in foods from the vegetable and starch/bread lists.

Sodium—A mineral needed by the body to maintain life, found mainly as a component of salt. Many individuals need to cut down the amount of sodium (and salt) they eat, to help control high blood pressure.

Starch—One of the two major types of carbohydrate. Foods consisting mainly of starch come from the starch/bread exchange list.

Sugar—One of the two major types of carbohydrate. Foods consisting mainly of simple sugars are those from the milk, vegetable, and fruit exchange lists. Other simple sugars include common table sugar and the sugar alcohols (sorbitol, mannitol, etc.)

Triglycerides—A fat normally present in the blood which is made from food. Excess weight, or consuming too much fat, alcohol, and sugar may increase the blood triglycerides to an unacceptably high level.

Vitamins—Substances found in food; needed in small amounts to assist in body processes and functions. These include vitamins A, D, E, the B-complex, C, and K.

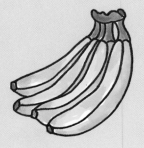

᛫ INDEX ᛫

puffed cereals, 7
pumpkin seeds, 21

R

rabbit, 11
radishes, 22
raisins, 17
raisin bread, unfrosted, 7
raspberries, 17
rhubarb, 22
rice, white or brown, 7
ricotta cheese, 12
romaine lettuce, 22
rutabaga, 15
rye crisp, 8

S

saccharin, 22
salad dressings, 21
salad dressings,
    low-calorie, 22
salami, 13
salmon, 12
salt pork, 21
saltine crackers, 8
sardines, 11
sauerkraut, 15
sausage, 13
scallops, 11
seeds, most kinds, 21
sherbet, 24
shredded wheat, 7
shrimp, 11
skim milk cheeses, 12
snack chips, 24

soups: chunky, cream,
    vegetable, 23
soy sauce, 22
spaghetti, 23
spareribs, 13
spices, 22
spinach, cooked, 15
spinach, raw, 22
squash, summer, 15
squash, winter, 7
squirrel, 11
steak: flank, round,
    sirloin, 11
steak: cubed, Porterhouse,
    T-bone, 12
steak: USDA Prime cuts, 13
strawberries, 17
stuffing, bread, 8
sugar substitutes, 22
sunflower seeds, 21
Swiss cheese, 13

T

taco sauce, 22
taco shells, 8
tangerines, 17
tea, 22
tofu, 12
tomato, 15
tomato juice, 15
tonic water, sugar-free, 22
Triscuit®, 8
tuna, in water, 11
tuna, in oil, 12
turnips, 15
turkey, 11

V

vanilla extract, 22
veal: lean cuts, chops,
    roasts, 11

veal cutlets, 12
venison, 11
vinegar, 22

W

waffles, 8
walnuts, 21
Wasa® crackers, 8
water chestnuts, 15
watermelon, 17
wheat germ, 7
whipped topping, 22
white breads, 7
whole-wheat breads, 7
whole-wheat crackers, 8
wine, in cooking, 22
Worcestershire sauce, 22

Y

yams, 7
yogurt, 19

Z

zucchini, 15